Letters Along My Journey

My Experience with Cancer and Chemotherapy

Angeline Graser

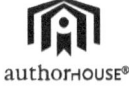

authorHOUSE®

AuthorHouse™
1663 Liberty Drive
Bloomington, IN 47403
www.authorhouse.com
Phone: 1-800-839-8640

First published by AuthorHouse 6/14/2010

ISBN: 978-1-4490-9592-5 (e)
ISBN: 978-1-4490-9590-1 (sc)
ISBN: 978-1-4490-9591-8 (hc)

Library of Congress Control Number: 2010908522

Printed in the United States of America
Bloomington, Indiana

This book is printed on acid-free paper.

Cover Design by: www.Last7studios.com

Photography by: www.ChrisGraser.com

This is for my son, Christopher
With all my love, Mom

Testimonials

I consider it a blessing to have a friend like Angeline. Her journal of experiences going through this ordeal is one of courage and faith. She was informed and, for the most part, was able to maintain her sense of humor and strength of character. I believe this book would be of great value to anyone going through chemotherapy, and I admire her for sharing her "deepest, darkest valley" in her life to help others and their families.

I believe that prayer was one of the most important factors, along with her faith, in helping her survive this tremendous ordeal. This has opened my eyes to the fact that the human spirit is an amazing gift if it is focused on prayer and faith.

I love you, Angeline, and am proud to be a friend.

Ellie Hartmann
Lake Worth, FL

This remarkable book will be a tremendous gift to anyone who has cancer, or to their families and friends. It is uplifting, inspiring, humorous, and honest, and really tells it like it is. I learned a lot while reading it. The words "cancer" and "chemotherapy" have to be two of the scariest words around. At least after reading this, I know what to look for to protect myself and how to help my friends that sadly have to go through it. We all have to take one day at a time to live our lives, but this shows us how to make the most of each day no matter what we are going through. God bless everyone who is helpful to those who are going through cancer.

Judy Thomas
Sayner, WI

Table of Contents

Introduction

My name is Angeline; I was a healthy woman until I was diagnosed with stage III ovarian cancer. Talk about a punch in the stomach! I remember first hearing the words "ovarian cancer" when I heard on the news about Gilda Radner's death. I remember thinking, "What a tragic loss for us." Hearing about all the symptoms that quietly mimic other bodily complaints we may have and choose to ignore must have stuck in my subconscious. My subconscious gently nudged me to talk with my doctor when something just wasn't right.

You can research information on the various cancers out on the Web and get overwhelmed with the knowledge, facts, and figures out there. I did not know what to expect physically and mentally. People just don't like talking about their pain, how long it lasts, and how they are handling it. So people suffer in silence while our surrounding family members and potential caregivers stand helplessly by, wondering what is going on. Those who read my letters told me my story should be told as it helped them tremendously. I wasn't asking for sympathy, just understanding. I wanted anyone associated with a cancer patient to feel empowered not helpless. I wanted them to know that doing little things make a big difference in a cancer patient's journey. So, here are my personal letters to family and friends as I walked my journey.

Prologue

After my hysterectomy, ovarian cancer diagnosis, and subsequent chemotherapy sessions, I continued to go in to work when I was physically able. I needed to stay productive and still have some kind of income coming in until the chemotherapy shut me down. I applied for the Family Medical Leave Act (FMLA) coverage through my employer and used all my paid time off (PTO) benefits I had accrued. I always planned for the unexpected, thus purchasing short-term and long-term disability through work, and I am sure glad that I did. It gave me one less thing to think about. Believe me, just because I had cancer did not mean I could stop paying the bills or worrying about where the money would be coming from. I also had purchased a cancer insurance policy years ago just in case, which also helped financially.

I wanted to feel as normal as I could during this phase of my life. I also needed a moral boost from my co-workers. To show my appreciation of their support, I gave each who wanted to wear one an ovarian cancer pin I was able to obtain. My son still has his on the cap he wears almost every day. My son still wears the teal ovarian cancer rubber bracelet I gave him. Every time it wears out, he replaces it. Physically being around people who are so concerned helps a person along the lonely road of cancer.

I soon realized I needed to document my journey, as I told my story to everyone who asked, "How are you feeling?" and "How is chemotherapy going?" I wouldn't always remember all the memorable moments, or I would end up doing an abbreviated version. Everyone was concerned and starving for information, as this topic and what a person experiences along the way was new to most of them. After they read one or more of my letters, I would get comments like "My husband never said a word while being treated for his cancer. I had no idea what he was going through," or "I have a friend just diagnosed with cancer and scared. This will help both of us get through this time in our lives. Thank you so much." So, this book is for the cancer patient, caregivers, family, relatives, friends, co-workers—anyone touched by cancer in his or her life. I know every cancer type gets different types of treatments with a whole different set of side effects. But just knowing what could be possibly going on with the person with cancer can greatly affect how you will treat and respond to him or her. And if nothing else, pray a little harder for them. Enjoy.

1

The Discovery Of Ovarian Cancer

Late January, 2008

Hi everyone, I just wanted to let you know what has been happening to me lately.

It all started with my going for my annual Pap check-up in November. I mentioned a spotting problem that just started. You see, for my fiftieth birthday, Mother Nature decided to stop my monthly periods. Hallelujah! So, my doctor, Francisco A. Estevez, MD, ABFP, checked me out. I always like it when the doctor tells you to relax while your butt is nearly off the table after having to slide down until he tells you to stop; your feet are in the cold metal stirrups (why don't they give you socks to keep

1

your feet warm?); you have a gel-covered, latex-gloved finger doing you know what while at the same time he is pushing down on your stomach, feeling for something. (Men, have you ever tried this? What, you would be too embarrassed?) Ah ha! He agreed something was going on. He ordered an ultrasound to see just what was happening. Upon receiving the results—tuberous mass in the uterus, eleven-centimeter cyst on the right ovary, and a small cyst on the left—he set up an appointment with a gynecologic oncology doctor by the name of James Fiorica, MD, of the First Physicians Group of Sarasota, whom he knows is one of the best. He sent my results to him before my first appointment. On my first appointment at the gynecologic oncology physician's office in December, his nurse practitioner, Maggi Tabano, ARNP, took a sample of the uterus tissue to send in for a pathology report. I was told they could not touch the cyst and possibly disrupt anything because of its size. Upon Dr. Fiorica receiving the results, my appointment was scheduled, and he explained what I needed done: a hysterectomy. The results showed the uterus tissue was benign but the cysts needed to be removed and sent out for further testing.

I had a hysterectomy January 21. My son, Christopher, thought it was quite apropos, as it was his birthday. Dr Fiorica removed every conceivable part in that area, fourteen bits and pieces to be exact. I donated all remaining tissue not needed for the pathology report to H. Lee Moffitt Cancer Center & Research Institute, Inc., for use on further cancer research. My gynecologic oncologist is affiliated with the H. Lee Moffitt Cancer Center & Research Institute, Inc. I am more than glad to help further research for new treatments and finding a cure. The consent form I signed, titled "Total Cancer Care: A Partnership with High Risk and/or Diagnosed Cancer Patients for Life," gave me a good incentive also. I was informed that sometimes, cancer patients can feel as if they have been "singled out" by this disease. Yet, in the state of Florida alone, nearly 100,000 cases of cancer are found each year. This is mind boggling. Then stop and think, if each state has a similar average number of new cancer cases each year, just how many people in the United States alone are getting diagnosed with cancer each year. Unbelievable! Cancer is a tough disease to treat because a lot of cancers look alike. If they study the medical histories, clinical records, blood, and tissues from thousands of patients, they might find better ways of treating cancer. They think there is a lot of information stored in your blood and in your tumor that can change the way they treat cancer in the future. They hope this study will answer many questions that doctors have not been able to answer before. There are more than two hundred types of cancer, and they hope this study will help physicians decide what type, how much risk, and the best treatment for any cancer. The procedures of this study entail answering a set of questions regarding past medical history, diet, risk factors, and any kind of treatments you may have had in the past. They then study your answers and review your medical records to see what you and other cancer patients have in common; store excess tissue removed at the time of your surgery; and collect tumor samples at the time of your diagnostic biopsy, additional blood samples at the time your doctor orders your laboratory tests, and urine samples in the preoperative period prior to tumor resection. All of these procedures are part of what you are already having done by doctor's orders, so you are not going out of your way to do it. If research on my donated tissue, blood, and urine may help to discover future treatments for a cancer like mine, or maybe a cure, then why would I think twice about participating? The survival rate of ovarian cancer is so poor; I just had to do my part. That is who I am.

Healing from this surgery is quite different from the ones I have had in the past. The outside body feels pretty good, other than tenderness on the left side of the incision. Dr. Fiorica said that this is internal bruising from all the work that he did inside. This tenderness will heal with time. I can be awake and about for between four to six hours at a time. But then, my body requires sleep for sometimes up to eighteen hours. The inside heals at a different rate than the outside, a much longer, slower process. It needs all the energy it can get to do its thing. So, I have learned to rest often during the day, and I don't mean catnaps. I put my head down and am out for a solid three to four hours sometimes. I also cannot sit for long periods of time because of where the work was done. I walk around the house or lay in bed listening to CDs. Slowly I am increasing my sit-up time so as not to tax my energy.

The pathology report on all the parts removed was not what I expected. The ovaries and some of the surrounding tissue came back malignant with stage III ovarian cancer. *Wow!* No known cause and no known cure. *What?* The good news was that it had not spread to the lymph nodes, but chemotherapy is still needed. I guess this is good news. If chemotherapy can be considered good news! An appointment was made with a doctor specializing in cancer treatments that Dr. Fiorica trusted and is friends with. I trusted his choice of the cancer doctor to send me to as I figured he most likely would not be friends with a doctor who did not do good work. Also, I do not have any family or friends who have had ovarian cancer, so I could not procure any physician references. When time is of the essence, checking the yellow pages for a doctor specializing in cancer treatments and going for the unknown when the mind is whirling with the word "cancer" did not seem like a feasible option. I trusted my doctor the first time, so I figured the best would send me to the best. I have always been a trusting person, and God has never let me down.

I went to the Florida Cancer Specialists' clinic and met with one of the doctors, Brian T. Berry, MD, who specialize in hematology and medical oncology. He explained my stage of ovarian cancer. They do not know why some women get ovarian cancer. I do not have a family history to indicate a genetic predisposition to it. Therapy is based on the stage of the cancer. The gynecologic oncologist removed all the cancer he could find. The minimal residual cancer left is what we are treating now. The cancer can spread to any part of the body due to the normal pelvic washing of the body. We will be doing a CT scan of all the major organs to determine if the cancer has spread and to have a baseline for future scans.

I have a slow/aggressive type of cancer. It is slow, as it takes its time sauntering around looking for a new home before getting down to serious business and only likes moving to familiar areas to grow. Thus, it went from one ovary and its related parts to the other. But, once established, it gets aggressive. For example: the cyst on the right ovary started out at eleven centimeters in November and came out a little over twelve centimeters. The left ovary's small cyst grew to six centimeters in two months. This also makes chemotherapy tricky. Chemotherapy can only destroy fully developed cancer cells, not the cells in the incubation stage. So, after my last chemotherapy treatment, I will have to have periodic CT scans and possible further chemotherapy if cancer reappears. I will be starting, in the near future, three-hour IV drips consisting of Taxol (Paclitaxel) and Paraplatin (Carboplatin), along with nausea medicine. This will occur every twenty-one days for six sessions. The goal is to prevent the cancer from reappearing or delaying it.

You know the TV commercials you see from the pharmaceutical companies regarding their new product and the list of possible side effects it may cause. Well, the two drugs I will be taking have some pretty scary side effects that have occurred in various users. Taxol (Paclitaxel) has caused reddening of the skin; itching; fever; rapid or troubled breathing; chest pain; fast heart rate; abnormal heart rhythms; very low or increased blood pressure; sudden swelling; hives; rash; decreased white blood cells, which can make me more prone to infections; lower numbers of red blood cells leading to tiredness; shortness of breath; paleness; dizziness upon standing; complete hair loss; joint and muscle pain; inflammation and soreness; sores in the mouth area; numbness; or tingling or burning in the hands and/or feet, which can indicate nerve damage. Paraplatin (Carboplatin) has many of the same side effects mentioned above, along with decreased platelets making one prone to easy bleeding and bruising, nausea and vomiting, ringing in the ears, hearing loss, vision changes, changes in taste and confusion, diarrhea, loss of appetite, weight loss, constipation, and stomach pain. Good grief! With all of these to watch for, it makes one afraid to leave the house. Also, it makes one wonder what is worse: cancer or the drugs you have to take. I need to eat as regularly as I can, get plenty of rest, and do some light exercises, stay away from stress and anxiety (Right! How is one not to think about all that might happen to you with those side effects?), and keep thinking positively. Okay, folks, keep praying for me. I am going to need a lot of strength to get through this.

You fashion-conscious ladies who stay current with the fashion magazines, I will need your help on how to wear scarves fashionably (pictures will help). Nancy, who I did not know had a form of cancer and is from the office of one of my clients I work with, is sending me some of the scarves and hats she used after her various treatments. I will be getting with the American Cancer Society, and they will show me how to use makeup so as not to scare anyone when all the hair is gone on my face. I wonder if men who get cancer no longer have to shave every day. And do they have to draw eyebrows on for vanity reasons? Too bad it isn't October; I always wanted to go as Uncle Fester for Halloween. After my first chemotherapy session, we will shave my hair off. Everyone says this is the smartest way for two reasons: it puts me in control of my recovery and eliminates globs of hair lying around or clogging drains when it does start to fall out in patches.

Last but not least, survival rate: Depending on what you read, stage III ovarian cancer has a 19 percent to 47 percent survival rate if it does not spread to other organs or lie in wait. For the small number of women who are fortunate enough to have their cancer diagnosed before it has spread beyond the ovary, the chance for cure is 85 percent to 90 percent. However, for the majority of women in whom the disease has spread beyond the ovary, the chance of living for five years after the diagnosis is between 20 percent and 25 percent. This has Christopher, my son, scared. After he talked with a friend and her mother, who is an occupational doctor, about my condition, he came by me sobbing, not wanting me to die, to be around to see him graduate, get married, and have children. I was doing pretty well until then. We have to take one day at a time and make the most of each moment together. My son will try to go with me to all doctor appointments and chemotherapy sessions, stay well informed, and keep an eye on me. I have purchased from the health food store some energy powder to make drinks to help me get through the bad days when energy starts lagging. Buy individual packets, if possible, to taste first before buying larger quantities. The first kind I purchased was not to my palate's liking no matter what I added to it. Now, everything depends on how my body accepts the chemotherapy, how healthy I can stay, how positive I can remain, and how many prayers the Lord is bombarded with.

Once I have the results of the CT scan and have had my first chemotherapy session, I will let you know what it was like. I will try to stay upbeat.

Thanks for all the prayers. I will need them for some time to come.

Love to all, Angeline

2

First Chemotherapy Session With Effects

Early February, 2008

Hi to all of you, I am back with an update on the next phase of my recovery.

On Thursday, February 7, I went for a CT scan of my major body organs. I got two bottles of banana-flavored barium sulfate to drink. Banana favored, ha! It only smelled banana flavored. The nurse who gave it to me said to drink it through a straw so it doesn't touch the taste buds. So, I found the fattest straw I had, put it all the way back to my throat, and drank the stuff in two gulps. It did work that way. I only got the taste when I pulled the straw out. I then quickly proceeded to brush my teeth and mouth. I had to fast for four hours, so this was my lunch. Ugh! I couldn't wait to get real food in me when the test was finished. They give you an IV so they can insert the dye for the test. When injecting the dye, they stated I would feel some tingling. The only thing I felt was my butt getting very warm. It is amazing how fast this stuff goes through your veins. I got injected twice, so I had hot buns twice. The sliding table you get to lie on is only twenty inches wide. It is not the most comfortable thing to lie on and not made for people of ample girth like me. When you move into the machine, you are told to hold your breath until told again to breathe. They must think that everyone has a lung capacity like an opera singer. It was a very long time to hold one's breathe, and I did take the deepest one I could. I almost didn't make it. And I had to do this four times. What fun!

On Tuesday, February 12, I had an appointment with Dr. Berry at the cancer clinic to go over the CT results. These are the findings: heart and arteries are in great shape; lungs and thyroid gland are also in good shape, with only a small nodule present on the left lung and thyroid (nothing serious, just need to be watched for growth); liver is normal with several variously sized cysts present, which will be watched also; spleen, gallbladder, pancreas, and kidneys are all normal. The only worrisome news was a small tumor found on the right front of the brain, which will require an MRI for further characterization. I told the doctor that my grandmother and one of her sisters died from brain tumors. So, I am now scheduled for the MRI on Friday, February 15. I figure by the time I get done with all this testing, I will know what is going on inside my body and what to keep an eye on.

I gave myself a Valentine's present, my first chemotherapy treatment. My son, Christopher, drove me as I had to be there by 10:00 AM. First thing they do is blood work to check red and white blood cells, as well as platelets. I am starting out with the following numbers: red blood cells, 13.3 for HGB (good range is 12.0 to 16.0) and 41.2 for HCT (good range is 37.0 to 47.0); white blood cells, 5.3 (good range is 4.0 to 10.0); and platelets, 326 (good range is 140 to 440); all of which are good numbers. Just remember, I just finished having surgery, so the numbers are down a bit. Once the results are in, you are taken to the chemotherapy room. The cancer center I went to for my chemotherapy has its chemotherapy room divided into three U-shaped sections with two nurses assigned to each section. Most nurses in this room have been in this field of work for ten or more years. So, as my nurse Pam stated, "We know what we are talking about, can explain the drugs being used, and have see almost all reaction types." It was good comfort for someone who has butterflies doing their dance in her stomach. I guess I am a little nervous! Now, get this: Pam comes back and asks if I am pressed for time. I say no and why? It seems my insurance company has denied their request to give me chemotherapy, which this particular insurance company has been doing a lot of lately, per Pam. Now, the insurance company wants preauthorization on all the drugs they are going to use in the procedure. They couldn't tell us that since they gave the okay for the chemotherapy session? And you have to administer these drugs before the chemotherapy drip starts. It gives me real confidence knowing someone at a desk knows what is best for me and not my doctor. It took almost one hour to get everything approved, and in the future, if they stop one drug and want to replace it with a different drug, you got it, preauthorization for the new drug. So, while I was waiting, Pam said I could nibble on the Valentine treats brought in by the other nurses. Oh my gosh, there were hot meatballs, chips and onion dip, salsa and chips, a sausage and cheese platter with a variety of crackers, deviled eggs (not as good as Linda's from work), Valentine cookies, and cupcakes. This is in addition to the normal snacks they have on hand for the patients to munch on as well as beverages of almost all types. (Sorry, no alcohol.) I do not have much of an appetite right now. Before the procedure starts, I am given a sojourn bear to provide comfort, inspiration, and support through my journey by making it bearable. My bear's name is Shelly (good omen: at the company I work for, I have a client contact person named Shelly and a client called Shelley's) and the bear is made from butterfly material. Boy, did she hit the mark when she picked the bear out for me. Each unique bear is handmade with love by caring volunteers. The group that makes the ones for this cancer center is the Ladies of Tree Lakes. I am also given a red tote from Lilly Oncology, which contains a note pad with pen; a water bottle, which will be great for mixing my energy drinks; and a small pouch containing Biotene products: mouthwash, toothpaste, and gum. This product helps with dry mouth or mouth sores as a result of the chemotherapy. My son's friend's mom recommended I get some of this product as it does work. I am now prepared.

Now, I get the drugs. Pam informs me that every session will take five hours. What happened to the three hours the doctor told me? It seems the prep drugs take an hour to drip, the primary chemotherapy drug drips for three hours, and the secondary chemotherapy drug drips for one hour. My son decides to go home and tells me to call when I am finished. They use a vein in your hand, as the bags of drugs given are hung on a three-legged metal tree like you see in hospitals for IVs or transfusions. This allows you to get up and move around to snack or go to the bathroom. Just remember, they are putting all these liquids in you, and they have to go somewhere. Okay, now let's find a vein. Pam found a good one in my left hand. Guess what, the needle hit a nodule in the vein. I mean the needle would not budge, and it hurt! She thought maybe it was scar tissue, but I don't normally take needles in the hand. She then proceeded to find a good vein in the arm just above the wrist and struck pay dirt on the first try. The first hour I get steroids, nausea medicine, Benadryl (diphenhydramine), and one other drug, which I don't remember, all at one time. Guess what, one of the drugs gave me restless legs. I could not sit still or get comfortable in the chair. Pam said this sometimes happens and was waiting for preauthorization for the drug they could give me to calm my legs down. This took about a half an hour to get, which was a very long time when you can't sit still and your legs want to keep moving. What a strange sensation! Upon inserting the drug into the IV line, the restlessness rapidly disappeared. Then I became very sleepy. I only got two chapters read in the book I brought along. Next, I got the serious drugs. Every hour or so, I got up to go to the bathroom and get myself a snack. I did eat my peanut butter and banana sandwich, which I brought from home before doing any snacking. Overall, they pumped one liter of liquids in me. I leave not knowing what will be happening in my body next. I am given information on the drugs they gave me. And the nurse recommends I start taking one hundred milligrams of the vitamin B6 three times a day to help prevent nerve damage to my fingertips and toes. I do have this amount of B6 in my daily vitamin. I stopped at the health food store on the way home and bought a bottle of the vitamin B6. I will then only have to take the supplement twice a day. The one I found at the health food store was on sale and is timed released. So I have that base covered.

Upon leaving the clinic, I get a blue piece of paper with the common side effects of chemotherapy. Nausea: take the prescribed anti-nausea medications for which I have a prescription, stay away from alcohol for twenty-four hours, and do not eat fried or spicy food on the day you receive chemotherapy or any time you are nauseated; stay away from milk or milk products while nauseated.

I don't know about you, but if I am nauseated, food and drink never even enter into my mind to try. Diarrhea: avoid milk, dairy products, citrus juices, and fried or fatty foods. If I am nauseated, I shouldn't worry about having diarrhea; drink plenty of clear liquids; take Imodium AD (loperamide) as directed on the sheet. If the diarrhea persists after twenty-four hours, call the office. I think I would be totally exhausted at the end of twenty-four hours. But there is one bright spot; I would not be gaining any weight! Constipation: take a stool softener, which you can buy over the counter; take milk of magnesia (I remember my grandmother taking this stuff); this next one is good, prune juice and butter. Mix a half cup of prune juice with one tablespoon of butter and melt; drink very warm at least two times daily. Okay, now, prune juice is difficult enough to drink cold, but warm? Ugh! But if I am desperate, I guess I would even try this. And last, mucositis (sores or redness inside the mouth): use baking soda and salt (one teaspoon to eight ounces of water); use Biotene mouth products, which I now have; but never use over-the-counter mouthwashes. It makes sense; who wants the alcohol burning an already sensitive mouth? Avoid citrus juices and spicy foods—do some people enjoy pain? Here is another good one: use Hurricane spray. Yes, there is such a product. I looked it up. It is 20 percent Benzocaine, which anesthetizes the affected area. Or you can use Ulcerease, which is an anesthetic mouth rinse. The knowledge of pharmaceutical products on the market is getting a little scary.

Friday, I awake a little tired and a little not quite myself. I have a 10:00 AM appointment for an MRI on my brain tumor. Christopher takes me, as he doesn't want me driving. The test takes a half an hour, and I get injected with more dye, but not the type that gives me hot buns. While I am having the MRI, Christopher went to my place of employment to pick up the Girl Scout cookies I ordered from Debbie in the benefits department. I enjoy the Girl Scout cookie time of year and will savor each bite this year. He enjoyed seeing everyone there and is instructed to have me call work more often with updates. I will try. Once home, I realize things are happening inside me. I start aching from head to toe; literally, every body part hurt. I had asked my doctor how chemotherapy would affect my arthritis. He said it would either make it feel really good or really bad. Of course, my body opted for door number two, dummy me! By Saturday morning, every inch of me hurts. I wish I had one of those Tempurpedic beds they advertise on TV. It hurts to lie in bed as well as to stand or sit. It is as if all the drugs spent Thursday evening and Friday looking for their best spots in my body. Then, come Friday evening, they exploded into action. I can actually feel what they are doing. My brain feels as if there are a lot of shorted wires crackling up there. My eyes ache, and when closed, it looks as if a strobe light show going on. All my joints are on fire. (I am typing this on Monday, as my fingers hurt too much over the weekend to use the computer.) So, I sat, walked, and lay down, trying to get comfortable. I did not get much sleep Friday or Saturday. By Sunday, the pain subsided from my upper body but is still in my legs. They ache to walk, and my ankles and feet are very tender. I cannot even spread my toes apart without a throb of pain. But the good part is I am able to sleep some Sunday night and even dream somewhat. Monday, I have a mild ache in the legs and am walking a little better, but not very fast yet.

I am telling this like it is, folks. This is not pretty. Please take ovarian cancer seriously and either go get tested or watch the silent signs and talk with your doctor for peace of mind. I would rather see you healthy than have to go through this. I am going to have to go every week to get my blood tested as the chemotherapy depletes the blood and platelet counts, which in turn will make me more susceptible to sickness and tiredness, as well as make me bleed easily when scratched.

Thanks for all the prayers and cards. I have prayer groups at three different churches praying for me. God is being bombarded. And Debbie, thanks for the gift of a beautiful cream-colored scarf and for all the information on where cancer patients can purchase scarves and hats along with all the nifty instructions on the various ways to tie scarves around the head. I am glad I will have time to practice; some of the versions are quite interesting. Trying these out should help distract the thoughts of pain and uplift my spirit.

Love to all, Angeline

3

Getting Ready For Second Chemotherapy Session

Mid-February, 2008

Hi everyone, here is my next installment of life with chemotherapy.

> Page 3: Those of us old enough to remember Paul Harvey's news at noon on Saturdays remember he always let you know what page he was reporting from. I can still hear his voice.

FACTS—OVARIAN CANCER

> All women are at risk.
> Ovarian cancer will be diagnosed in about one out of fifty-five women (approximately 1.8 percent).

Ovarian cancer counts for about 3 percent of all cancers in women.

Symptoms exist—they can be vague, but increase over time.

Early detection increase survival rate.

A Pap test *does not* detect ovarian cancer. It is a screening tool to detect cervical cancer.

SOME SYMPTOMS

Pelvic or abdominal pain or discomfort

Vague but persistent gastrointestinal upsets such as gas, nausea, indigestion

Frequency and/or urgency of urination in the absence of an infection

Unexplained weight gain or loss

Pelvic and/or abdominal swelling, bloating, and/or feeling of fullness

Ongoing unusual fatigue

Unexplained changes in bowel habits

If symptoms persist for more than two weeks, consult your physician.

While the symptoms of ovarian cancer (particularly in the early states) are often not acute or intense, and are often not taken seriously because they are similar to other female bodily complaints, they are not silent; they whisper, so **LISTEN**. If any of these ovarian cancer signs are experienced almost every day and persist for weeks, they could be an early warning of ovarian cancer and should be brought to your doctor's attention. Over 70 percent of all women with ovarian cancer will not be diagnosed until the disease has spread beyond the ovary. Women experiencing continued symptoms of ovarian cancer should have a combination of ovarian cancer tests that include pelvic examination, vaginal ultrasound, and a CA125 test.

This information was found on The Gilda Radner Familial Ovarian Cancer Registry, The American Cancer Society, and Ovarian Cancer-Mayo Clinic sites.

On Sunday, February 17, we shaved my head. Christopher took me outside, as I didn't want this mess in the house, and used his shaver. He didn't go all the way to the scalp, but close enough. He was a little scared but had a blast. He never thought he would see his mother bald. As soon as he was finished with mine, he did his head. When done, and after sweeping up all the hair (no, I didn't leave it lying around for the birds to use to make nests with), we went back into the house to do the final shaving of the scalp. This was done by a friend of my son's, also named Chris. He has been shaving his head since high school and has it down pat. He wanted to make sure my son didn't nick my scalp. He lathered my scalp and used one of those little pink BIC shavers. What a weird sensation. When it was all done, I touched my scalp and could not feel it. It was in the state of shook. I had no trouble sleeping with my bald head, but I didn't realize how much heat your head discharges. My pillows get very warm. I also discovered that when the air conditioning comes on at night, the head cools off really fast. I had to sleep with a cap on. Driving in the car with the windows open feels so good with none of the hair blowing in one's face. Now, I have to put sunscreen on my head to keep it from burning. I have been told it is no fun to get a sunburn on the scalp (how would you put your head on the pillow?) and have it peel. Ugh, that must look awful, as if you were molting or something.

I went to my first blood testing after chemotherapy on Thursday, February 21: my red blood count showed a very little decrease; my white blood count and platelets were just fine. I had a list of questions to ask the doctor, seeing as I now had gone through the first session. All my concerns were the possible side effects in different versions, and he recommended I keep doing this after every session. The doctor did prescribe a pain pill to handle the second and third day of discomfort, seeing as four Advil did nothing for me. They want me to be comfortable so the body can rest without more things to worry about. The nurse did recommend I get my eyes checked to make sure they are healthy, seeing as they ached and chemotherapy does accelerate some conditions. I told her I had scheduled an appointment for Thursday, February 28, and this would provide peace of mind. The nurse also mentioned that six to ten days after the treatment is the lowest time for your body. I didn't know that! That explains why I was so tired driving to the appointment when I got up at 9:00 AM to be there by 10:00 AM. It was the seventh day.

I will have to be extra careful to get plenty of rest during this time frame and not be around anyone who may be getting sick or is sick. *Beware*: when I come back in to work, I am going to have a large can of Lysol to keep my area protected. I promise not to use too much of it so we don't gag from the odor.

Ginny gave me tickets to see the stage production of *Jersey Boys* at the Tampa Bay Performing Arts Center on Sunday, February 24, for the 2:00 PM performance. Oh my gosh, it was spectacular! The songs brought back so many memories; I found myself crying. Even Christopher was blown away by the performance. I just had to buy the CD to play in the car on the way home and visualize the performance on the stage, which I am sure I will be doing all through my recovery process. It felt good to get out other than going to church and doctor appointments.

Christopher took off from work the week of February 25 through March 1 to spend time with me. He will just be going to classes instead of classes and work. Monday, he had various errands to run and wanted me along with him. It was fun in the car with the windows open and the wind blowing through my scalp. (Bet you thought I was going to say "through my hair.") I did have a scarf on, but it still felt good. My body was getting tired, and I did not realize it. Come Tuesday, I slept until 3:00 PM, which really shocked me. I felt fine those two days, but I guess my body hasn't caught up with the rest of me yet. I will have to slow down for a while.

I went to see my gynecologic oncology doctor on Thursday, February 28, and got a clean bill of health. Everything is healing just fine, but the doctor recommends no heavy lifting for a while yet as the insides are still in the healing process. Next, I went for my weekly blood work; all three counts they are monitoring are down. I was surprised that a third of my platelets have not replenished themselves yet. Normally, they do it in one or two days. It also explains why my body is tiring more often, and my brain just doesn't comprehend yet. I guess I will have to increase naps and food consumption of the nutritional foods to help the blood counts. My doctor was out of the office this week, so I do not have an update on the brain scan yet, but I did get to talk with his nurse. She took my vital signs, listened to my breathing, reviewed the lab studies with me, updated my chart, and took any questions she could not answer to give to the doctor. She told me that either she or another doctor at the clinic would be seeing me at these weekly blood work sessions. My regularly assigned doctor would definitely see me the day of the chemotherapy. This place is very busy. Last was the eye doctor. Pressure in the eyes is back in the good range, so I do not need the drops I have been taking any more. (These were for a condition prior to the cancer diagnosis.) Overall, my eyes are healthy. They will check my eyes again in two months after my last chemotherapy session to see if anything changes. I hope not.

It looks as though I will be back to work on Monday, March 3, but I don't think it will be full days. I will have to get my stamina up for my next chemotherapy session on Thursday, March 6. Where did twenty-one days go? Keep those prayers coming; they are helping me stay strong.

Love to all, Angeline

4

Second Chemotherapy Session With Effects

Early March, 2008

Salutations everyone, I am back with my experience of the second chemotherapy session.

You know how you dread something, an argument with a friend or having a tooth pulled, knowing there will be pain? That is how it is with me for the second chemotherapy session. I know what to expect, and it isn't nice. After the argument or having the tooth pulled, you know the pain will go away, and you will be back to normal. But going to chemotherapy, you know the pain will be the same or greater or lesser; your body is take a beating and try to recover, and then you hit it with another session of chemotherapy. You don't want to think about it, but the thought creeps up when you least expect it. I have placed my trust in the Lord, but human nature as it is, I still worry. I shouldn't; He has His arms wrapped around me. Why can't I trust as a little child does? It takes a lot of strength, prayers, support, and encouragement to get through that door. I now have a deeper respect for anyone who has walked this route, time and time again.

I also believe your inside body knows what you are doing to it and resents it. My veins never hurt when a needle was stuck into them for blood work before, but now they balk and cry out. How do I know? I used to be an apheresis donor, giving platelets for cancer and leukemia patients. I would go every month and have a needle stuck in both arms for a two-and-a-half-hour period. Ok, so I watched a good movie to keep my mind off of it, but the veins never squawked. While living in North Carolina, I was matched with a patient and gave every week. Same thing, no problems, the veins cooperated. Well, almost. I was watching the first *Die Hard* movie at one session, as the guys in the room picked it out. I was so upset with the violence that my veins kept closing up, sending the machine into spasms. Once they removed the headphones so I couldn't hear the movie, everything calmed down, and I finished the session. I did watch the movie in silence and complained when Bruce Willis didn't kill the bad guy the first time when he had a chance. Everyone just laughed.

So, I decided to help psych myself up by buying a new nightgown, a pink one. I figure you always feel so special when wearing something new. So, after the Thursday session of chemotherapy, I will wear the new nightgown for the three or four rough days and tell myself how I am pampering myself and being a lady of leisure. If it works, I will continue this method until all sessions are finished, and I can wear the nightgown every day as I get stronger! I will probably have to come up with additional pick-me-ups to add to each session. Maybe for next time, I will buy myself a new set of sheets, the kind with the high thread count! I am told they make you feel as if you are sleeping on a cloud.

A former co-worker of mine, Cathy Snyder, stopped by on Saturday, March 1, and dropped off a beautiful, soft, crocheted comfort shawl. She belongs to the Hands to Hearts Handcrafters of the First Baptist Church of Bradenton, FL. The card inside read, "May this comfort shawl, that has been handmade with prayers interwoven in the stitches, bring you comfort. As you wrap it around you, may our Creator God, the Cradle of Comfort, the Keeper of Deep Places, the Enfolder of all Life, cradle, keep and enfold you with hope, joy, peace, love and healing." I love wrapping it around my shoulders, as it is so soft, and will take it with me to my chemotherapy session on Thursday, so there will be plenty of love going into me along with the chemicals. Also, a current co-worker, Muriel, gave me a crocheted "comfort ghan." Her note read that she is a member of an Internet-based volunteer group called Heartmade Blessings. They make "comfort ghans" when they hear that someone needs a little comfort, no matter what the reason. She received a pattern book at Christmas and has been crocheting up a storm. Once home after my first session, whenever I was sitting, I would be chilled and have to get a blanket. Now, I have this beautiful lap-sized comfort ghan to use, and the color scheme goes with my furniture. God must have given her some insight when picking out the colors to do this one.

I went back to work on Monday, March 3. I felt good and was ready. As the day wore on (I only worked four hours in the morning), I felt the tiredness creep in, and I was hardly doing anything. Was I ever so glad to get home! I made myself a bowl of homemade soup, which I received from Aline. She had Barney whip up a batch of homemade vegetable soup and brought it over one Saturday. It is *sooooo* good. I put some in the freezer for future use when I am too tired to cook. Anyway, after eating, I lay down for my nap and slept until 6:00 PM, when my mother called to see how I was doing. The nap felt so good. Tuesday and Wednesday were a little bit better at work, but Wednesday, I did more payrolls than on Tuesday, so I was ready for my nap when I got home.

Thursday, March 6, came in as a cloudy and cool sixty-two-degree day. My chauffeur for the day was the Rev. Shirley Whitaker, pastor of the Emmanuel Worship Center, Inc. She is also the sister of Alice, one of my son's co-workers. She said she had the whole day free and wanted to spend it with me. I could just feel the love wrapped around me. Shirley loves to talk and kept conversation going from the time she picked me up until I went in for the chemotherapy drip. While sitting in the waiting room for me to get my blood work done, Shirley met two ladies that she worked with twenty years ago at a day care center. One had her husband in for his drip, and the other lady was getting a drip. So, Shirley's conversation kept up with both of them until they both left. What are the odds of a meeting like this? God's hand was definitely in this one. My red and white blood counts, along with my platelets, all went up. The doctor was very pleased with this, along with my not having any serious reactions to the first chemotherapy session, just the arthritis flare-up and the normal side effects. I asked about the brain tumor scan, and the cancer doctor said there is a small tumor, which they think may be benign. They want to wait and see after all the chemotherapy sessions what the next MRI shows as far as growth or reduction. My drip went very well. I didn't need the strong prep drugs, just half the dose. So, the tiredness was not as extreme, and the restless legs were mild. Walking to the bathroom every hour calmed them down. Listening to the audio book I brought along this time also helped. The time just flew by. Shirley left around 2:30 PM, and Christopher came to pick me up at 3:45 PM. I had just finished all my drips—what good timing! On the way out there was a box of knitted and crocheted hats along with scarves (not there the last time I came) with a note on the wall to take one or two. They are gifts with prayers of encouragement from Hats of Hope, a ministry of Abundant Life Church on Proctor Road in Sarasota. I picked out two scarves; one was reversible, to compliment my wardrobe. I was sure blessed with prayers this chemotherapy session, God's answer to my concern on how it might go. What wonderful signs. Driving home, I felt tired, so we had a light supper, and I went to bed early to let the chemicals get acquainted with the first residents. I hope they get along and not misbehave and throw a sorority toga party!

It was a restless night; my legs would not calm down until around 2:00 AM. I then fell into a deep sleep and slept on and off all day Friday. When I woke I would eat something light, as I knew I would be falling back asleep. The stomach was not quite settled from the chemotherapy, so I took a nausea pill to help it get along. Saturday came in with the arthritic knee dancing to "Hail, Hail, the Gang's All Here" from around 3:00 AM. Most of the day, I just lay around, taking a single Lortab (Hydrocodone Bitartrate/Acetaminophen) to help combat the knee pain; it didn't do much, though. I kept myself wrapped in my comfort ghan and comfort shawl. That felt really good. Then, around 6:00 PM, the pain just exploded inside, from top to bottom, like fireworks on the Fourth of July. Here, I thought it was going to be a light session from what I was experiencing all day! Now, I moved up to two Lortab (Hydrocodone Bitartrate/Acetaminophen) so I could get some rest, which is what I did all day Sunday and Monday. These cold fronts better stop coming at the same time I do my chemotherapy sessions. I get hit with a double dose of arthritis, one from the weather and the other from the chemotherapy. My legs are taking a beating this session, with aches from the hip down to the sole, thus making it hard to get comfortable when trying to sleep, stand, or sit. Walking is a little shaky from the pain. My taste buds changed this time; everything tastes blah, which makes it hard to keep drinking water when it tastes so bad. I have tried adding some flavors to the water, a little improvement but not much. I do have an open bottle of wine in the refrigerator but, of course, the Lortab (Hydrocodone Bitartrate/Acetaminophen) bottle states alcohol will intensify the drowsiness. I don't dare take a chance with no one home. Shucks! Tuesday brought the pain down to my knees and below. I hope it is on the way out of my system. Tuesday evening brought another pain flare-up, just what I needed.

WARNING:
READING MATERIAL MAY NOT
BE SUITABLE FOR ALL.
DO NOT BE EATING DURING DISCUSSION OF
CONSTIPATION, HEMORRHOIDS,
AND THE FINGER.

I discovered I was constipated from taking the Lortab (Hydrocodone Bitartrate/Acetaminophen). This was part of the side effects; I didn't read far enough down the list. It didn't help my disposition. I am now trying prune juice, which isn't so bad if ice cold (yeah right!), but hot? Forget it, stool softeners, suppositories, and Preparation H because my hemorrhoids are now flared up and hurt. The flare-up of pain in my hands and the headache had me walking the floor Tuesday night. I didn't want to take the Lortab (Hydrocodone Bitartrate/Acetaminophen) and cause any more constipation problems, and Advil just wasn't doing the trick. I guess I finally fell asleep from exhaustion. Poor Christopher didn't know what to do to help me, other than to stay up with me and try to be of some comfort. Wednesday came in with exhaustion. I went to see my family doctor, Dr. Estevez, about my constipation and hemorrhoid problem. Unfortunately, I couldn't get in until the end of the day. I told his nurse, Rita, that not every family has a child happy because his or her mother has finally had a BM, but it sure hurt. She just started laughing, as she has known us for a long time. When the doctor came in, I told him what was going on. I had to get up on the table and lay on my side. He stuck his lubricated finger inside, and the salve was cool to the touch. I sighed, and he apologized. I told him it felt good, as it really is hot down there because it felt as though I was throwing flames. I don't know, but it must have struck him and the nurse as funny, as they laughed so hard they had tears. He said I had torn the inside hemorrhoids open, which were very angry and letting me know about it, as well as swollen and bleeding. He gave me a prescription for a cream to use both inside and out every time I go. Now, I get to use the finger. I guess I better cut the nail short on that finger. I don't need to tear anything else open. I will treasure this prescription, as my co-pay was fifty dollars. He also told me to take a stool softener when taking Lortab (Hydrocodone Bitartrate/Acetaminophen) so this problem does not occur again. Oh yeah, I will follow those instructions religiously. Thursday brought pain relief, much needed sleep, and fiber eating, so I could keep things moving.

I am planning to go back to work part time on Monday, March 17. I should be more myself by then. I might even make it a whole week but will not push it if the body squawks. Thanks for all the prayers. I now have a group of bikers praying for me. A fellow employee is a biker and ministers to his group. He told them about me, and I am now on their prayer list. When I found out about that, it put a smile on my face. I wonder what God thinks about that!

Love to all, Angeline

5

Third Chemotherapy Session With Effects

Late March, 2008

Hi everyone, chemotherapy session number three is coming up.

I forgot to mention in my last update my hair dilemma. As you know, I shaved it off before it fell out. What I didn't know and could not find in my rereading of side effects was that it actually hurts falling out. Those startled roots did not know what hit them, and they were balking to have to leave their home. The first chemotherapy session only started to kill the hair roots. So, after we shaved my head, the hair continued to grow, but at a much slower rate. I had this sixteenth of an inch of growth on my head. Christopher always patted me on the head when he walked by. All of a sudden, those love taps were hurting. Now, how do I remove this growth from my head? Shaving again would only remove the upper growth and leave the dead roots in my scalp to hurt. Christopher suggested I use a lint roller, but I did not have one. I tried Scotch tape, but my scalp was too oily for the hair to stick, a problem I have always had. Packing tape's adhesive is too abrasive and would probably remove some skin along with the hair. So, I tried the old standby, duct tape, and it worked quite well. I gave Christopher the honors. When pulled off, and it was the coolest sensation, the tape was dark with all the short hairs. So now, all I have left of my hair are those wiry white hairs that are refusing to leave quite yet. They are pure white, which I hope is the color when my hair grows out. My father had pure white hair until the day he died. What a wonderful crown of glory to have when done with all the chemotherapy

The morning of my third chemotherapy session started out a wonderful fifty-eight degrees and with sunny skies. That is a whole lot better than a cold front coming through. My driver for today was Carol Cox, a co-worker who only works three days a week and is off on Thursdays and Fridays. My session was at 9:00 AM, so Carol was promptly at my home at 8:25 AM. Unfortunately, she had to wait while I finished packing my bag lunch, peanut butter and banana sandwich with raspberry white tea; my iPod with headphones to listen to the next audio book; a hard-covered book just in case the iPod fails (five hours is a long time to stare at the ceiling or nurses—no, I am not of that predisposition!); my trusty notebook; and my comfort shawl. She dropped me off and would return at 2:00 PM, when I would be finished. My blood work was excellent as my white blood count almost doubled from the previous week. (It must have been those wonderful liver sausage sandwiches and coleslaw made with red wine vinaigrette I was enjoying for lunch each day.) My nurse this time was Marcy. She started the drip using a vein in my left hand. I am not too happy about using my hand, but she did find one vein that cooperated. She explained to me why they start in the hand. Once they use a vein, they can never go below the previous injection site. They always have to move up. This made sense of why, the first time I went and they chose a vein in my left hand, it did not work. It was the same vein used in the hospital during my surgery. So, my body threw up a wall to block any further intrusion, letting us know we needed to move up the street, so to speak, if we wanted to use the vein any more. Also, a vein can become traumatized from the chemicals and needs time to heal itself. That explains why one of the veins in the left arm felt as if I had a series of small pebbles in it, which have since dissipated. The next session will be done in the right arm to give the left a rest. I only had restless legs for about two hours this time and not as forcefully. I enjoyed some wonderful donut holes from Dunkin Donuts and homemade raisin cookies made by another patient's wife. Time flew by with the audio book I was listening to, and before I knew it, my time was almost up. Carol arrived promptly at 2:00 PM, but I was still going to be on the drip for another ten minutes. She was able to sit with me, as the chair next to me was vacant. By the time I put my things away and had a short chat with Carol, I was finished. I took it easy the rest of the day and slept well.

Friday, I awoke feeling tired but no pain yet, but that would end soon enough. By evening's end, the left knee was warming up its vocal cords to Queen's "We Will Rock You." I could feel every stomp. Saturday came in loud and clear. Every part of my body ached, from the top of my head to the bottom of my feet, and this included places that did not hurt the first or second time. The head was tender, so placing it on a pillow was not an easy task. I had to find the right spot with the least amount of pressure. The eyes preferred the dark to light. The neck ached, so keeping the head upright was dismissed and lying flat was opted for. The ache in the shoulders radiated straight to the fingertips. It hurt to hold a glass or use silverware to eat. No, I stayed respectable and did not lick my plate clean. My appetite was dull, so not much food was required, and again, water tasted terrible. I still do not have my full taste buds back yet. My ribs hurt as well as the lower back, pelvis area, hips, calves, and feet. I have the strangest sensation with my toes: inside, they feel very cold, but outside, they are warm. So, I keep putting my slipper socks on and off. How am I to rest when every part of me hurts to stand, sit, or lie? Try finding a soothing spot when there is none to be found! I just got into a position and stayed there until the pain increased, then on to a new position. It is scary lying there and feeling the chemicals working and wondering how they know where all to go. But then again, chemotherapy is a free spirit, going where it pleases, not caring what it destroys in its path, over and over again. It must sense the previous visitors and figures they must have missed something. The pain had me in tears. I wanted a hug but knew it would hurt. I took my pain medication, but because I was hurting in so many places, it could only do so much. Probably, when it hit my stomach, it didn't know where to go first to relieve the pain. I did not abuse it and just took the recommended dosage along with the stool softener each time. What I really needed was for the pain to stop. I slept some every hour. You see, I have a grandfather's clock, which chimes every quarter hour, and I always heard the hour chime as well as the quarter hours most times. Added to the pain, nausea crept in with dry heaves. I wasn't eating much, so there wasn't much to come out, thus the ribs hurt more for trying. Then there were the cold chills and hot flashes. Oh my gosh! I would have the blanket up to my neck to stop the chills, then the hot flashes came over me, like the continual ocean waves on a shore, and I could feel the heat radiating from my body. Pam from work calls them her private summers. Mine definitely were not Florida summers. Mine were more like the oppressive Serengeti summers. I never experienced hot flashes like this when I had all my normal body parts. I am told these are part of the chemotherapy aftermath. If I was living up north,

I would be definitely melting snow. This session kept me flat on my back for three days. I did try sitting up but only lasted two hours before the tears came, so I decided it wasn't worth the effort. And to think I have three more sessions of this to look forward to! Tuesday, I was able to get out of bed for a while and actually sit for a period of time. I won't take that simple pleasure for granted anymore; that is for sure.

I received two surprises in the mail on Tuesday. One was a package from the American Heritage Life Insurance Company, Allstate Workplace Division. (I have a cancer policy through them.) The package contained a letter from David A. Bird, CLU, ChFC, President, and a book titled *Chicken Soup for the Surviving Soul: 101 Healing Stories about Those Who Have Survived Cancer."* His letter read that he had just been informed about my cancer claim and just recently became aware of the enclosed book and thought I might appreciate the inspiring stories from those who have shared my experience. He sincerely hoped it would bring me comfort, strength, and encouragement. Wow! Whether he actually wrote the letter really doesn't matter; just taking the time to send both to me put a bright spot in my gloomy mood, and, of course, I cried. I immediately sat down and sent a thank you note explaining my reaction to their thoughtfulness.

I cried a second time when I read a letter from my aunt Rosemary in Wisconsin. She was wondering if I could send a set of my letters to my second cousin, who was recently diagnosed with cancer and is just devastated. As I keep the tone light yet informative, his wife and children, if not him, would better understand what he will be going through and better understand how to deal with their emotions, support, and encouragement. Boy is he going to get a fat letter with all five of my letters. I, who rarely speak but rather listen, was being asked to help someone with my words. This just blew me away.

Guess what? Wednesday came in with me feeling a little better and getting diarrhea! Yes, it was another side effect of chemotherapy. So now, I have added Imodium AD (loperamide) Advanced to my table of medications. My poor body is trying out every side effect. I wish it would remember what it was like to be normal and work to try to get that way. Of course, this has added to my exhaustion.

Thursday, I was back for blood work. My counts are down, but that is to be expected. I mentioned I was not doing any recuperative sleeping at night and was given a prescription for a sleeping pill to be used very carefully and only as needed. I haven't picked it up from the pharmacy yet but will be interested in what my co-pay will be for this one. I had taken in paperwork for the doctor at the cancer clinic to update my status for my short-term disability. The insurance company only used my gynecologic oncology doctor's report, which stated I could work full time as of March 17. Thus, they have stopped payments until they reevaluate my claim. I explained to him I only work four hours a day; any longer, I get really tired. The doctor mentioned that exhaustion would only get worse as the chemotherapy sessions continue, and four hours a day may become too much. I told him I understood, but it was nice being with my fellow co-workers for a change, but I would take one day at a time. I just have to watch myself, with Aline's (a co-worker) gentle supervision, of course, and be careful. Now, it is time to put my feet up and read some more stories in my book. And keep those prayers coming.

Love to all, Angeline

6

Fourth Chemotherapy Session With Effects

Mid-April, 2008

I am back and just realized that I am half finished with my chemotherapy sessions. *Yeah!*

By the tone of my last report, I was pretty down from the reactions I went through. But I had cheering up, with a week's visit from my brother, Gregory Black, who lives in Boulder City, Nevada, and a day visit from my cousin, Mark Wager, who lives in Hollywood, Florida. And while working on this report, I had a good friend, Gen Miller, who lives in the park where I live, stop by with homemade chicken noodle soup—mmh, mmh good. And another lady from church, Patricia Grzanich, brought me homemade applesauce and apple butter. Now, these kinds of delicious surprises I like.

After my first chemotherapy session, I started experiencing a mild shortness of breath. After the second chemotherapy session, the shortness of breath came after any task I did, like walking from the kitchen to my bedroom or folding towels and putting them away. I just had to sit down and slow the breathing down. One knows when his or her breathing is not right, and I mentioned this to the doctor, who ordered a chest X-ray. It came back with my lungs being clear, no fluid buildup, and no pneumonia. Even though my red blood count is close to the low end of acceptable, my body is requiring more than I can produce right now. The red blood cells carry oxygen to cells in the body, and if the count is low, the organs in your body don't get enough oxygen. The two tests they perform on every blood draw show them two things: first, how much protein is in the cells, as protein carries oxygen in the blood; and second, how much of your blood is made up of red blood cells. What I can do to help is get enough rest, move slowly (no power walking or even a pace swifter than normal) from place to place, and eat foods rich in iron. Okay, I think I need a grease board in my dining room so I can list all the foods I should be eating and figure out how to get them all in each day. Iron-rich foods are meats (I love red meat!), chicken, and dark green vegetables (when I have been able to eat, I have been eating lots of green beans, but I better change the lettuce to spinach in the salads), along with foods high in vitamin C. I have been eating oranges and just bought some granny smith apples. So, I am eating right, just not enough every day. I will definitely have to improve the eating skills, but I refuse to put foods in a blender and make a drink out of them. I don't care what Jack LaLanne says when he is demonstrating his food blender; I like to taste each food!

Another count they monitor is the white blood cells, which help the body fight off illness and infections. I must guard against outside sources of germs from people, pets, and standing water. (I guess I won't be jumping in puddles for a while!) So, if you cough or sneeze around me, you get Lysoled! I must keep my hands and mouth clean. That means washing my hands often and rinsing my mouth after meals as well as morning and bedtime. No cuts or scratches or chapped lips are allowed. And your lips do get chapped. I have salve on them at all times. No open door for any type of germs. The other counts they monitor are the platelets, which are blood cells that help blood clot. So, I have to be careful not to nick or cut myself by mistake, gently blow my nose and brush my teeth (I had to replace my firm bristle toothbrush with a soft one for the time being; I do like the scrubbing feeling with the firm brush versus the swooshing of the soft one), prevent hard bowel movements (I learned my lesson regarding this one), and possibly avoid having sex. Yes, if the platelet count is very low, the doctor may suggest that sex be avoided. This will help prevent any internal bruising. Well, I don't have to worry about that one, either!

I went for my weekly Thursday blood draw and discovered that my white blood cell count is very low. I have to stay away from people and germs, which means I cannot go back to work until the count goes up. It was suggested I rest and do whatever I can to get the count up for the chemotherapy session next Thursday. This is really important because the chemotherapy does hit the white blood cells pretty hard, and I don't want all the cells to be killed. I need them.

With my brother Gregory here, he was able to take me and pick me up from my fourth chemotherapy session. My nurse this time is Tulia. Yes, with a T not a J. This session, we started using the right hand for the injection site. It was a little tough for the needle to go in, but we got there. Being right handed made it interesting going to the bathroom! Before the session, I spoke to the doctor about all the pain I had the last session, which lasted a good three days. He gave me a prescription for Dexamethasone, a corticosteroid, which will help with the pain. I take it twice a day with food. He said this is one of the drugs they give me before the chemotherapy is inserted to help with pain. It explains why Thursday and Friday I have no pain, then get hit on Saturday because it is all out of my system. Possible side effects from this drug are difficulty sleeping (this explains why I am now taking sleeping pills to stop the staring at the ceiling through the night); nervousness; increased appetite (well, I know I don't have this problem, as everything tastes like metal right now, and I mean everything, so the thought of eating is not a pleasant one); indigestion; nausea (which

I have had a lot of lately, so I am taking the nausea pills more often); chronic back pain (this explains why while sitting, my lower back ached, and I could not get comfortable in any chair or couch); headaches (I had one for three days until I stopped this medicine); muscle aches or weakness (my shoulder blades hurt so badly I thought I had gotten a massage from a WWE wrestler); fever; cold; prolonged sore throat; vision changes (my eye ached, so I kept the rooms darkened from the light or just covered my eyes altogether—thank goodness for audio books!); swelling of feet, hands, or legs; black, tarry stools (believe me, with all the medication you have to take along with the chemotherapy, everything comes out either black or green. It is as if you are rotting from the inside for a while. Eventually, it gets back to normal); mood, mental, or personality changes (heck, with all I am going through, this should not be a side effect; it should be normal!); and seizures and skin growths (you've got to be kidding!). I took this pill on Saturday through Monday, which helped a lot. By Tuesday evening, my stomach hurt so badly, that I stopped all medicine and took Pepto-Bismol to coat and soothe my stomach. I needed the irritation to stop, and it worked! I told the nurse practitioner about this, and I now have to take Prilosec OTC every day to keep the irritation at bay. If this pill would not have worked, I would have had to go back and have a system flush IV, which would quickly flush all the chemicals from my system, thus cutting down on the time they had in my body to kill the cancer. I'm glad the pills worked.

The worst of the pain settled in my legs, with my calves hurting and the toes on my feet going numb. Try standing in the shower and balancing without feeling your toes. I sure am glad I have two grab bars in the shower. For sitting, I put a pillow under my legs to give the calves some softness. I also had some tingling in the fingers of both hands. When I went for my blood work, I had a long discussion with the nurse practitioner about all my symptoms. She explained I am getting the highest chemotherapy dose allowed for my type of cancer and is concerned with my feet and hands. She will discuss this with the doctor and see if they can lower the dosage for the next two sessions, so nerve damage does not become permanent. I told her I am taking the B6 vitamin as they suggested, but I was told it sometimes is not as effective as it should be. Great! The fatigue is increasing with my tiring often after doing an activity. She said this is normal and not to fight it or be ashamed of it. Just listen to my body and take care of it. With all it is going through, it is struggling to survive. Besides my body, my spirit was overwhelmed this session. That is why this update is a week late. I could not get my mind focused to sit at the computer and type. It just wanted to curl up in a cocoon and hibernate for while, thinking of nothing. As no one can help with the physical or mental pain your body is going through, you feel like an island being washed with the waves of a hurricane, waiting for the constant pounding to pass. You know in time it will, but the waiting takes its toll. Not deep sleeping didn't help either. I was tossing and turning with the series of hot flashes and chills. But now, with the sleeping pills and soothing music to sleep by, the mornings are more refreshed, and the spirit seems to like this.

I went again this morning for my weekly blood draw. Results were not good. All counts are dangerously low, which means staying away from all people either at church, the store, restaurants, and work. One of the most serious side effects of strong chemotherapy is a low white blood cell count. This condition is referred to as Neutropenia. Without a sufficient white blood cell count, the body cannot fight infections, and I may be at risk for developing severe and potentially life-threatening complications. Being the bright rays of sunshine that they are, the nurses told me that if I get an infection now, it would kill me, as I have nothing to fight it off. Thank you very much. Oh, and did I know that the residual chemicals of the chemotherapy can stay in my body up to two years before totally dissipating? I can't wait for my next visit! Maybe I should go all dressed in black for mourning the lack of joy they have. They mean well, but all this information never comes with a positive side.

I now have to take shots of Neupogen (Filgrastim), which is a white blood cell booster. It works by stimulating the growth of neutrophils, a type of infection-fighting white blood cell. It signals the bone marrow to make more neutrophils. Symptoms include abdominal or shoulder pain, rash, and shortness of breath, wheezing, dizziness due to a drop in blood pressure, swelling around the mouth or eyes, fast pulse, or sweating. Okay, I already have shortness of breath and sweating from the hot flashes. The nurse said I will feel a lot of bone pain as we are forcing the bone marrow to work double time to increase its count. She said to take plenty of Advil to help with the pain. This should be really interesting. It is a good thing I only have to take two shots for now. I wonder if I can sip on some Bailey's Irish Cream to help me relax and lift my spirits. Why didn't I think of this sooner! Keep me in those prayers. They sure are helping.

Love to all, Angeline

7

Fifth Chemotherapy Session With Effects And Near Death Experience

Early May, 2008

Hi everyone,

Boy, that chilled Bailey's Irish Cream sure was good. I had a bottle chilling since Christmas. It's too bad it wasn't a bigger size! I thought this was going to be a short update, but I had a near death experience, so put your feet up.

The Neupogen shots weren't bad, but the after effects were surprising. After the first shot on Thursday, I got very tired, so I had to lie down only to wake up sore all over. I had to take four Advil to ease the discomfort. I learned my lesson after the second shot on Friday; I took the Advil before I went to lie down. They knocked me out for four hours each time. Saturday, I ached a little but could handle it. I went to bed Saturday night and woke up at noon on Monday. I did get up to go to the bathroom, and Christopher got me up Sunday at 10:00 PM to drink some Gatorade to replenish my electrolytes. I just couldn't keep my eyes open. I placed a call to my doctor Monday afternoon to see if this was normal or if we should be worried. I was informed that I have a war going on in my body, and the Neupogen added a new fighting front. Thus, my body is getting so overworked at healing that it needed to shut down, and I listened very well. I also need to keep a water bottle by my bed and drink every time I wake up to help flush my system. I guess I will be peeing a lot more also! This sure is one way to get a lot of rest.

The day of the fifth chemotherapy session, the doctor was running an hour late. I have to see the doctor first to confirm the treatment for the day. Seeing as all my numbers improved and I still have the numbness in my toes, he decided to stop the Taxol (Paclitaxel) this session as it is causing the numbness. We need to get the nerve endings in my feet back to normal so there is no permanent damage. Stopping the Taxol (Paclitaxel) also cut three hours off my session, as this is the longest drip. Surprisingly, there was no usual pain by Sunday, but something settled in my lower back. I moved slowly Sunday, but by Monday, I could hardly stand or sit. I spent Monday through Wednesday flat on my back, only sitting to eat. I tried Advil, Lortab (Hydrocodone Bitartrate/Acetaminophen), and Icy Hot medicated patches, but nothing relieved the pain. The best solution was a heating pad. I would stay on it for ten minutes, and then cool down while napping (not really good when you are having hot flashes—you have to take showers twice a day!). Christopher noticed that my hands are shaking a little. Okay, this is a whole new set of experiences.

When I went for my regular blood work, all the counts have come up but are still too low. Does that make sense? I have to take another two shots of Neupogen this week to build up for the next chemotherapy session. You know, when they give statistics that state how many hours a person sleeps in his or her lifetime, I think they should do a separate one for people with cancer. Otherwise, with all the sleeping I am doing now, I will never have to sleep again when I get in my seventies and eighties. I wonder if my body knows this. I better start having long talks with it when this is all done. I don't want any surprises down the road! I also mentioned to the doctor about the persistent back pain, so he ordered a bone scan just to see if the cancer had moved into the bone. The scan came back negative, very good news.

I now want to give you my observations on who developed this poison I have to take, which is administered by a licensed physician and approved by the insurance company. A man! Sorry, but that is how I feel about it right now! My reasons are these: Men hate to go bald, so why not let women see what it is like? Men hate to shave their faces every morning, so let the facial hair all fall off and stop growing awhile. It would be interesting to see how men draw eyebrows on! And it also proves a man did the developing, as they did not compensate for us menopausal women who are blessed with the extra facial hair growth. Come on now, you all have seen *My Big Fat Greek Wedding*, right? There is the scene where the mother of the bride is getting dressed, and her best friend is using tweezers on her face. I am talking about the stubborn chin hairs, which, for me, grow out white and hard as a nail and unbelievably fast. Now you don't see them; now you do. As you are brushing your teeth, you take a closer look in the mirror and ah ha, there they stand at attention. It is always the day you are running late that ten popped out overnight, or so it seems. If I ever got stranded on an island, I could use them for nails. These hairs are still growing, and I still have to pluck them. It's not fair! I have enough to worry about. Now, I think this is where he lost control in the development process. I will give men my condolences for all the chest hair that falls out; that must really deflate their egos. Yes, down there is smooth as a baby's bottom. But why is my leg hair still growing? I would like a reprieve from shaving also. Maybe I am one whose leg hair is on the stubborn side and refuses to fall out. Or maybe, for men, it doesn't fall out. Oh my, I might have male leg genes! I will never know.

This is where my update was going to end, but then came the near death experience. I had no symptoms on Saturday when I went to bed. Sunday morning, I woke up and proceeded to walk to the kitchen. By the time I got there, I could hardly breathe and my heart was racing just like Big Brown, who ran the Preakness on Saturday. I thought I best lie back down and try to get the heart slowed down with some deep breathing, if I could. After a few minutes of trying, I had no luck, so I called the cancer doctor, Dr. Berry. The doctor on call said to go to the ER immediately. Man, I never saw my son fly out of bed so fast and get dressed when I told him to get up and take me to the ER. He was at the door waiting for me to get my shoes on. He drove a little over the speed limit and only passed on a double yellow line once. We took a lot of back roads to get to the hospital. We kept watching for a cop to pop out from somewhere to stop us. Since it was Sunday morning, the traffic was light as a lot of people were in church. Thus, no one's life was in jeopardy. When I got to the ER entrance, the nurse who takes all your vitals and medical history was standing at the door and walked me to her office. They were really slow. No one was sitting in the waiting room. They must have all been in church. After completing the information, I was wheeled to my ER room where all the monitoring machines were attached and blood taken. In no time, my family doctor, Dr. Estevez, arrived. He informed me that my blood work indicated I was having a mild heart attack. He wanted some cardiac test to be run, but the hospital did not have a doctor on duty to read the results, so that had to be scratched for now. He also wanted a test run on my lungs to determine my breathing problem. He ordered a CT scan of my lungs, for which I was hurriedly taken to that room. Unfortunately, the needle site used in the ER room would not accept the dye for the CT scan. The machine shut down, saying there was a blockage. Great! A nurse had to be called in to remove the needle and find a new site on the other arm. (Here we go again.) Once that was completed, we tried the test again, and it worked. The results showed my family doctor that I had a massive clot on my right lung and a smaller one on my left lung. They immediately administered a drug that would start thinning my blood and prevent further clotting for now, thus giving my body the start time to begin dissolving the clot. They are also lowering my blood pressure so the heart won't work so hard to get enough oxygen to all my body parts. My family doctor said I was very lucky that I came in when I did. If I had waited any longer, I would have stopped breathing and died. *Wow*, what an eye opener! And to think I missed Sunday mass. I was doing a lot of praying to make up for it. We caught the clots as they were just developing. He explained it was like getting a bruise: you bump and hurt, then get black and blue, then turn yellow. I was at the bump stage. He also explained that the heart and lungs touch each other. Because the heart was racing so fast, it released some of its chemicals into my blood, thus projecting a false positive for a heart attack. I was not having a heart attack, some good news. Poor Christopher was trying to write down all the medical jargon my family doctor was saying so he could ask a friend to speak with her parents (both doctors) for a better understanding of what was happening.

Once somewhat stabilized, I was escorted to my room on the cardiac floor. They did not know if any damage was done to the heart by this episode, so they were not taking any chances. I was hooked up to my own portable EKG monitor, which I had to wear twenty-four hours a day every day, and told to stay in bed. I could only get up to go to the bathroom with an escort. You do not know how often you go to the bathroom until you have to call for assistance. I finally learned to go when a nurse or CNA was in the room, lessening the wait time. The next day, when all the doctors came in to see me and give me their versions of what was happening, I asked why there was a clot. Several factors were pointed out to me. First, I already experienced a clot in my right leg after my first hip replacement, which was dissolved, thus raising my chances. Second, I had ovarian cancer. Whoa, the possibility of getting blood clots was never mentioned by any doctor during the cancer process. I sure would have been asking more questions about this situation. Third, my activity level dropped significantly. Okay, chemotherapy makes one tired along with the Neupogen (Filgrastim) shots. You are not up to much physical activity, and if you can't keep your eyes open, one has a tendency to fall asleep. I was caught between a rock and a hard place on this one! Fourth, I had a second hip replaced. Okay, all my doctors knew I have had both hips replaced. It was part of all the questions I had to answer on the forms each doctor provided me with. Did no red flags go up for them to warn me? For now, I am put on injections of Lovenox (it is an anticoagulant therapy indicated to help reduce the risk of developing DVT, or deep vein thrombosis, which may lead to pulmonary embolism, PE) in my belly and an intravenous drip of nitroglycerin along with oxygen. Keeping those little nozzles in your nose is no easy task. And don't keep it on when eating. I nearly choked on my scrambled eggs as I inhaled the oxygen and eggs at the same time. They both went down the same pipe, thus creating a good coughing spell. My other question was how long it would take for the clots to dissolve. The response was weeks. They just don't go away as quickly as they formed. They must be similar to gaining weight: easy on, years to take off!

So, what is the future? My family doctor, Dr. Estevez, said I would be put on Coumadin (Warfarin Sodium Tablets, USP) for the rest of my life. For those of you not familiar with this medication, I will give a brief explanation. Coumadin (Warfarin Sodium Tablets, USP) is an anticoagulant medicine. It is used to lower the chance of blood clots forming in your body, such as in the legs and lungs, or causing a stroke or heart attack. It also can cause serious and life-threatening bleeding problems. If you cut yourself, it may take up to ten minutes for the bleeding to stop. And that is with constant pressure being applied. Your liver makes clotting factors that help the blood to clot and prevent bleeding. Coumadin (Warfarin Sodium Tablets, USP) blocks the formation of clotting proteins in the liver that are dependent on vitamin K. Most foods have a low amount of vitamin K, but those with the highest content are leafy green vegetables, such as kale, parsley, spinach, and turnip greens, as well as broccoli and Brussels sprouts. Eating these high vitamin K–content foods would interfere with the blood-thinning effects of Coumadin (Warfarin Sodium Tablets, USP). Drinking cranberry juice or eating cranberry products along with drinking alcohol should also be avoided as they can interact with Coumadin (Warfarin Sodium Tablets, USP) and affect your treatment and dose. What is meant by "treatment and dose"? You need to get a blood test as often as your health care provider determines to check for your response to Coumadin (Warfarin Sodium Tablets, USP). This blood test is called a PT/INR test. This test checks to see how fast your blood clots. Of course, we want it to be slow. Your doctor determines what your PT/INR number should be. (Mine should be between two and three. While in the hospital, mine was a one, clotting very fast.) Your doctor will then increase the dosage of Coumadin (Warfarin Sodium Tablets, USP) to slow down the clotting proteins or decrease the dosage to increase the clotting proteins. Some things that can change your PT/INR results are prescription drugs, many over-the-counter medications, herbal medicines, or botanicals and vitamins. Thus, you need to provide your doctor with a complete list of everything, and I mean everything, that you are taking or have in your medicine cabinet to take when needed. Tell your health care provider about any planned surgeries, medical or dental procedures, as the Coumadin (Warfarin Sodium Tablets, USP) may have to be stopped for a short time because of the bleeding factor. Okay, did you think we could end without possible side effects? I have to admit that these are not as bad as the cancer side effects. We have death of skin tissue called skin necrosis or gangrene, purple toes syndrome, allergic reactions, liver problems, low blood pressure, swelling, low red blood cells, paleness, fever, and rash. See, they are not so bad.

Next, my cancer doctor, Dr. Berry, comes in and says no, we are not going to do Coumadin (Warfarin Sodium Tablets, USP). He is the blood doctor, and I will follow his regiment, as this is his line of work. I will be giving myself shots of Fragmin (dalteparin sodium injection) every day for the rest of my life. This drug is easier to regulate in the system than Coumadin (Warfarin Sodium Tablets, USP). Shots??? I started shaking and got a little scared. I just cannot imagine giving myself shorts. This is going to take some strong self-motivation! He said it was no big deal. Yeah, right. Is he giving himself daily shots? I bet not. This medication is injected under the skin but not into a muscle. That is why the belly is chosen. It's a good thing I fit into the category where the commercial asks if you have excess belly fat. That is me. I have plenty of area to put the needle in. Now, I have to learn how to properly dispose of used syringes and needles. Do they sell the red hazard boxes? Yikes, now when asked by a doctor or nurse if I have ever used a needle, I will have to answer yes. The needle is very small and does not hurt going in. It does burn for a short period of time once the medicine is under the skin. Many of the side effects are similar to the cancer ones. All my vital signs are looking good, and I was able to slowly walk around the nurse's station with a walker and no heavy breathing resulted. My family doctor says I can go home. I was able to leave on Wednesday afternoon. Discharge paperwork takes time!

I did not know that when Christopher sent out his email regarding my hospitalization on Sunday evening to everyone at my office that he included my room's direct line phone number. That is why I was surprised to get a call from a friend in Tennessee. She said it was in his email. He just smiled when I asked him. He didn't want me to be lonely. It was nice to get some cards while in the hospital along with a basket of fragrant flowers from my place of employment, a huge edible fruit arrangement from the previous owners of the company I work for. (I'm glad I was going home the day it arrived. There wasn't a refrigerator large enough, other than in the main kitchen, to hold it. Not that the nurses weren't nice, but they changed every day. I wanted to totally enjoy the eating pleasure with my son.) And Doriana Beshaj, a former co-worker, stopped by with a vase of beautiful lilies. I don't know if they were store bought or from her garden. They were huge!

I now have a cardiologist and pulmonary doctor to add to my repertory of doctors. They both want to see me in the next few weeks. The cardiologist (he is a good-looking man and ranked number two in the state—not that my other doctors aren't bad to look at) wants to see if anything happened to the heart as we never did conduct any tests. He has me taking 325 mg of aspirin daily along with Atenolol and Altace (ramipril). Atenolol is a beta-blocker. This drug works by blocking the action of certain natural chemicals in your body, such as epinephrine, on the heart and blood vessels. This results in a lowering of the heart rate, blood pressure, and strain on the heart. Altace (ramipril) belongs to a group of medications called ACE inhibitors. It works by relaxing blood vessels, causing them to widen. Most of the side effects are similar to the cancer ones, but there were a few unique ones. Altace might change the color of my skin to yellow. Atenolol may change my coloring to blue. I might get a butterfly-shaped rash on my nose and cheeks and have unusual dreams. I told Christopher to watch if my coloring changes to green and if he sees butterfly shapes on my face.

As for my giving the shots of Fragmin (dalteparin sodium injection) to myself, I have to wait for the prescription to arrive. As this medicine is costly (without insurance, $1,980.00 for a thirty-day supply of 500cc, and I will be taking 1300cc), it was cheaper to do by mail: a $50.00 co-pay per month or a $100.00 co-pay for a ninety-day supply. Once it arrives, my doctor will train me in the procedure. I wanted Christopher to be a back-up, but he nearly passes out at the sight of a needle. My family doctor wants me to ask the cancer doctor if he thinks putting in a Greenfield filter would be helpful. It is inserted through the vagina and placed below the liver as an added precaution to inhibit blood clots in the lower half of the body. I have not heard the doctor's response, probably at the next and last chemotherapy session.

And you thought you had a rough week! Keep those prayers coming! I don't know what will be thrown at me next, but your prayers are sure giving me strength. Thanks so much.

Love to all, Angeline

8

*Sixth And Last Chemotherapy
Session With Effects*

Late May, 2008

Hi everyone. Well, here it is: the sixth and last chemotherapy session. Hurray!!!

I was hoping it could be a light one like the fifth session, but that was not my luck. The doctor said this one needed to be a full dose. I also asked him about the Greenfield filter; he has heard about it, but doesn't feel comfortable trying it at this time as he feels not enough research or documentation has been done on what its success rate is. There is not much left inside to fight back with, so the end results were really draining. Constipation, lack of appetite, numb toes, and shaking internally were the side effects this time, in addition to having the mind feeling muddled and not able to warm up, which is not like me. I had the house temperature at eighty degrees and had a blanket on. Thank goodness this has passed. It is a strange feeling to feel your insides shaking and not be able to control it. Am I subconsciously worried about something? It is amazing how we take for granted the workings of our insides to make our outsides feel so good. At least now, my body can start to rebuild and not be knocked down again. Remember, when I first started chemotherapy, I gave you my red and white blood cell counts, along with my platelet count. Well, here are my numbers now: red blood cell, HGB 11.7 (range is 12.0 to 16.0) and HCT 34.1 (range is 37.0 to 47.0); white blood cells, 4.2 (range is 4.2 to 10.0); and platelets, 175 (range is 140 to 440). I have a way to go to get them built up again.

The doctor also ordered a Neulasta shot. (Neulasta is a prescription medication called a white cell booster that helps your body produce more white blood cells to reduce your risk of infection. A sufficient white blood cell count may enable your doctor to administer chemotherapy according to their treatment schedule.) It does the same thing as the Neupogen shot, only at a slower speed. It takes a full two weeks to reach its full potential in boosting all the cells and platelets. The drawback is the body aches for one week, every part of you. And, of course, it costs more per shot, five thousand dollars. The clinic where I go for my treatments does some research on site and cannot figure out where the manufacturers came up with its cost for medications. Just unbelievable! No wonder insurance companies balk at new drugs. Yet, all the ads on TV tell you to talk with your doctor and see if this new drug is right for you. It would be nice if a drug could be produced that would work its magic with little or no side effects and be reasonably priced. When I went for my blood work the following week, my counts were up by one half, very good news. Now, these healthy cells have to continue to reproduce and attack the chemicals to get rid of them to make room for healthy growth.

I now have peach fuzz on my head. My hair looks as though it will be brown. It always amazed me when ever I mentioned having cancer, the first words out of everyone's mouths are that the hair will grow back and be oh so curly at first. That's great if you don't mind going bald, but that is not everyone's preference. Going bald did not bother me. But I know a lot of people whose hair is what makes them feel whole, who resent being told this. I guess we need to be a little more considerate of a person's feelings. It would be much better if the cancer patient brings up the hair situation. Thus, you can get a feel for the attitude he or she is presenting and either joke about it or say nothing at all. Hats, scarves, and wigs are great but don't make us feel whole like the real thing.

I now am on my own doing the daily Fragmin (dalteparin sodium injection) shots to keep my blood from clotting. Some days are good; others hurt. The insurance company never gave me a starter kit on how to administer the drug. I just watched the nurses administer it and followed them. I just received the kit from my doctor. The kit contained a video and DVD on how to self-inject Fragmin (dalteparin sodium injection), alcohol swabs, a Sharps container for syringe disposal, a guide about how to self-inject Fragmin (dalteparin sodium injection), and important safety information, all quite useful and valuable to know. When the Sharps container is full, I need to take it to the county health department to exchange for an empty one. A question arose as to the various sites I could use. I was told the site was the stomach fat, which I have plenty of. But according to the kit, besides the U-shaped area around the belly button, I can also use the upper outer side of the thigh and the upper outer part of the buttock. (This would be done by someone other than me. I don't think looking in a mirror would work to well!) I tried the outer side of the thigh and found the injection site bleeds a lot longer than the stomach area. I went through five extra large bandages even with applying pressure. And that was before even leaving the bathroom. Then, when I thought the bleeding had subsided, it started up again when I started walking. (I have thunder thighs, so that didn't help matters.) I sure made a mess with a pair of pants I had on. I decided the stomach area will be the safest area to use from now on. It sure would be embarrassing to have bleeding problems at work. As the insurance company will not fill the prescription on a monthly basis, I have to call every other week to request my supply for fourteen days. Thank goodness there isn't a co-pay for this medication. I have updated my calendar accordingly. Well, what do you know? I just received a call from the mail order pharmacy asking if I needed the refill request processed. They also advised that the insurance company reconsidered the thirty-day supply and granted it. So now, I just have to get a refill every thirty days, which they ship via UPS to my door.

This journey has been a demanding one. It is great that so many people are praying for me. There have been family members and friends that have been in constant contact, either by phone, email, or a card. Or those who have dropped off soup or just a little gift to remind me I was thought of. I look at all my cards every week, rereading each message for support.

I have developed a few thoughts on how to be supportive of a long-term sick person. Don't let them drop off your radar! Those powerful words, "you have mail," are just that, powerful, be it email or the good post office. I know I was surprised in the hospital when a card was dropped off on my tray. And it did put a smile on my face. Prayers are wonderful, but a sick person cannot touch a prayer at needed times. We need a tangible reminder now and then to know people still have us on their minds. Some days, we get lonely with only our thoughts for companions. And believe me, those thoughts sure can play tricks on you. Then, you might say, why doesn't the sick person reach out and make contact? We are dealing with the pain, the changes we are experiencing physically, the future outlook, and the mental challenges. Before we know it, a day, a week has flown by, or we are too consumed with our situation to think any further. I know going back to work has not even crept into my mind. Doing everything I have been told to do has been my top priority as well as listening to my body. The challenge has been to survive the attack on my body and my emotions. Sometimes, you do not want to disturb the sick person as he or she may be sleeping or not up to company or a phone call. If we are not up to it, we will let you know. But you have no idea what a one-minute conversation can do to one's spirits. It is also hard to relate to a person who sounds well and fine on the phone or in person. They can't be that sick! Unless we are hurting so badly, we are going to do our best to be uplifting. This is what we need to do for ourselves. Please keep in contact; you have no idea how important this is to our well-being.

I have two tests scheduled this week, one for the heart and the other for the lungs. The cardiologist's office is working with an imaging firm that approves all imaging tests for the insurance company. The cardiologist scheduled a two-part test of the heart but only got approval for one part of the test. We are still waiting for the final approval to move ahead. The lung tests are scheduled for Wednesday. I guess the unknown has been working on my conscious and subconscious minds. I want everything to be all right to be able to move forward. The doctor is also going to redo all the tests I had done before the treatment started to see what changes, if any, transpired. At least after these tests, there are no side effects.

Keep the prayers coming! I need all the positive energy to help the healing process along.

Love to all, Angeline

9

Working On The Road To Recovery From Ovarian Cancer

June, 2008

Hallelujah, the chemotherapy is over!!!

I feel just like James Brown sang, "I feel good." I just can't do his foot movements to the song yet. (Every time I read this line, I picture him dancing in my mind.) My blood work is looking good; all counts are going up slowly. The doctor is pleased with all the test results; nothing abnormal was indicated. My cancer count went from 289 at the start to 7 at the finish, a very good number. Yes! And it needs to stay that way for the rest of the follow-up visits every three months for now. Eventually, they will change to every six months, then every year thereafter. This applies to both the cancer doctor and the gynecologic oncologist, who I will now visit for the rest of my life. Stamina will take a time to build up. Trying to carry something while walking gets me puffing, the same as any substantial distance walking. I just keep trying a little more whenever I can. My eye doctor reported the same good results; nothing has changed.

While reading the book *Chicken Soup for the Surviving Soul: 101 Healing Stories about Those Who Have Survived Cancer*, I read an article by a scientist and professor of medicine named June Goodfield. She is British and a fellow of the Royal Society of Medicine who has devoted years of her life to the study of cancer. She believes that once the treatments are completed, a person needs a total change of scenery, someplace quiet and beautiful. In her experience, a drastic change in environment can trigger a change for the better. It made sense to me! I have been looking at the same walls for four months, fluctuating between feeling terrible some days and feeling on the mend on others. So, I decided to take a two-week vacation. My son and I flew first class to cut down on the number of people around me. We went to northern Wisconsin, a quiet and beautiful place, to stay with my girlfriend since sixth grade. Judy Thomas and her husband, Gale Thomas, were overjoyed that I decided to spend this time with them. Judy said that since she could not help me out during my chemotherapy, she was going to pamper me. We stayed in one of their rental apartments above their house. I could spend time with them whenever I felt like it, which turned out to be most of the time. I just slept in the apartment. She did stock the apartment with some audio books, very good chocolates, my favorite chips, and a twelve pack of my favorite beer. (She got all this information from my son.) She really wanted me to relax! The days were in the lower seventies and the nights in the upper forties, no humidity. What joy! I listened to loons (a type of water bird) call on the lake and whippoorwills (also a bird) cry at nightfall. I listened to the wind blowing through the pines. Unless you have heard that sound, it cannot be described. It is so soothing. We took a ride around Plum Lake, which they live on, with one of their neighbors on their pontoon boat. We saw two eagle nests, one of which had two young in it. Binoculars are wonderful. Smelling the water and feeling the spray as the boat went along was a joy I had forgotten. We left the house to get some ice cream one evening and saw a four-hundred-pound bear at the end of their driveway. He took one look at us, knew we were going for ice cream, and decided not to mess with two women on a mission. We watched a turtle bury her eggs for hatching. My girlfriend has her own ceramic business. She insisted I just had to make something to bring home as a reminder of my stay. I made a wind chime. The stay was wonderful and way too short. It was just what I needed, a pick-me-up for the mind and the soul. I cried when I left. I didn't realize I missed northern Wisconsin so much. I will always have a place to go back to.

I now have a release to come back to work as of August, working up to full time. Your prayers have helped tremendously but still keep them coming for a while yet.

Love to all, Angeline

Epilogue

It has been two years since my journey started. What a growing and sometimes painful experience! I am still cancer free with my number now at one. I am anxiously awaiting the six-year cancer free mark. The survival rate for stage III ovarian cancer is between two to five years. If I make it to six years, then I beat the odds and am truly a survivor. I am so thankful for all my family and friends who came to me in my time of need without being asked. I loved all the homemade foods, gifts, visits, and especially the prayers. Without the prayers, who knows where I would be now. I still reread all the cards and notes I received during my journey. The words do wonders for my soul.

I am up and around but not at full speed. Chemotherapy has a tendency to lower your energy level. I tire faster when doing things, so they take a little longer to get done. I can live with that. In some people, it also affects short-term memory mildly or severely. My son says he sometimes notices this in me. I think he is just pulling my leg as he probably thought he told me something but mentioned it to one of his friends instead. I still have nerve damage in my toes. They may or may not ever be normal. My son thinks I am a klutz but I say that when you are not feeling your toes, one has a tendency to get too close to objects, thus stubbing the toes. But for not having feeling in them, it sure hurts to stub them. As the company I worked for changed insurance carriers, I had to stop the Fragmin (dalteparin sodium injection). The new insurance carrier considered it a prescription and would not cover it under the medical plan. At ninety dollars for a month's supply, it was no longer in my budget. I get restless legs now and then and found that Hyland's Restful Legs relieves the symptoms, and I can sleep. My hair grew back a beautiful dark brown with a few grays joining the crowd. No, it did not come back curly, as everyone told me it would. I got straight hair! Dang, I was hoping to save money and not have to get permanents for curls! At first, I had some waves, but they disappeared when I got my first haircut to get some shape to it. Everyone says they like the new look and that I should leave it this way. They prefer it to the curls. Why didn't these people tell me this sooner? Just think of all the money I could have saved over the years by not getting permanents.

I hope you have gained some insight regarding the road a cancer patient may have to follow. And I hope that it has enhanced your feeling on how you will respond the next time you hear someone say, "I have cancer." And if nothing else, pray a little harder for them.

God bless, Angeline

Index

About The Author

Angeline Graser was born and raised in Wisconsin, and graduated from Our Lady of Mercy High School in Milwaukee, Wisconsin, in 1965. She worked in clerical, statistical, and administrative positions for insurance companies in Milwaukee, Wisconsin, and Raleigh, North Carolina. She moved to Florida in 1990 to become primary caregiver to her parents, George (deceased) and Dolores Black. She is a past president of the Council of Catholic Women and past assistant youth group leader at Our Lady Queen of Martyrs Catholic Church in Sarasota, Florida. Since she is passionate about the knowledge needed to confront ovarian cancer and chemotherapy, a book of her experiences was inevitable. She lives in Bradenton, Florida, with her son, Christopher, who owns his own Web design company, Last 7 Studios.

About The Book

What is your first thought when you hear the word "cancer"? It's probably not a good one. Cancer changes us: some of us for good, others for bad. Ovarian cancer changed me. I became stronger, determined, and empowered. From being a listener, I became a writer. This book is about my journey through chemotherapy. As I told my story to family and friends, I discovered that besides being concerned, they were starving for information. This topic and what a person is experiencing along the way was new to most of them. It changed the direction of my life and helped others to look at cancer from a new perspective. You'll laugh with me, maybe you'll cry, but hopefully, you'll become a wiser person.